I Can't Sleep, I'm Depressed, and I Don't Want a Prescription

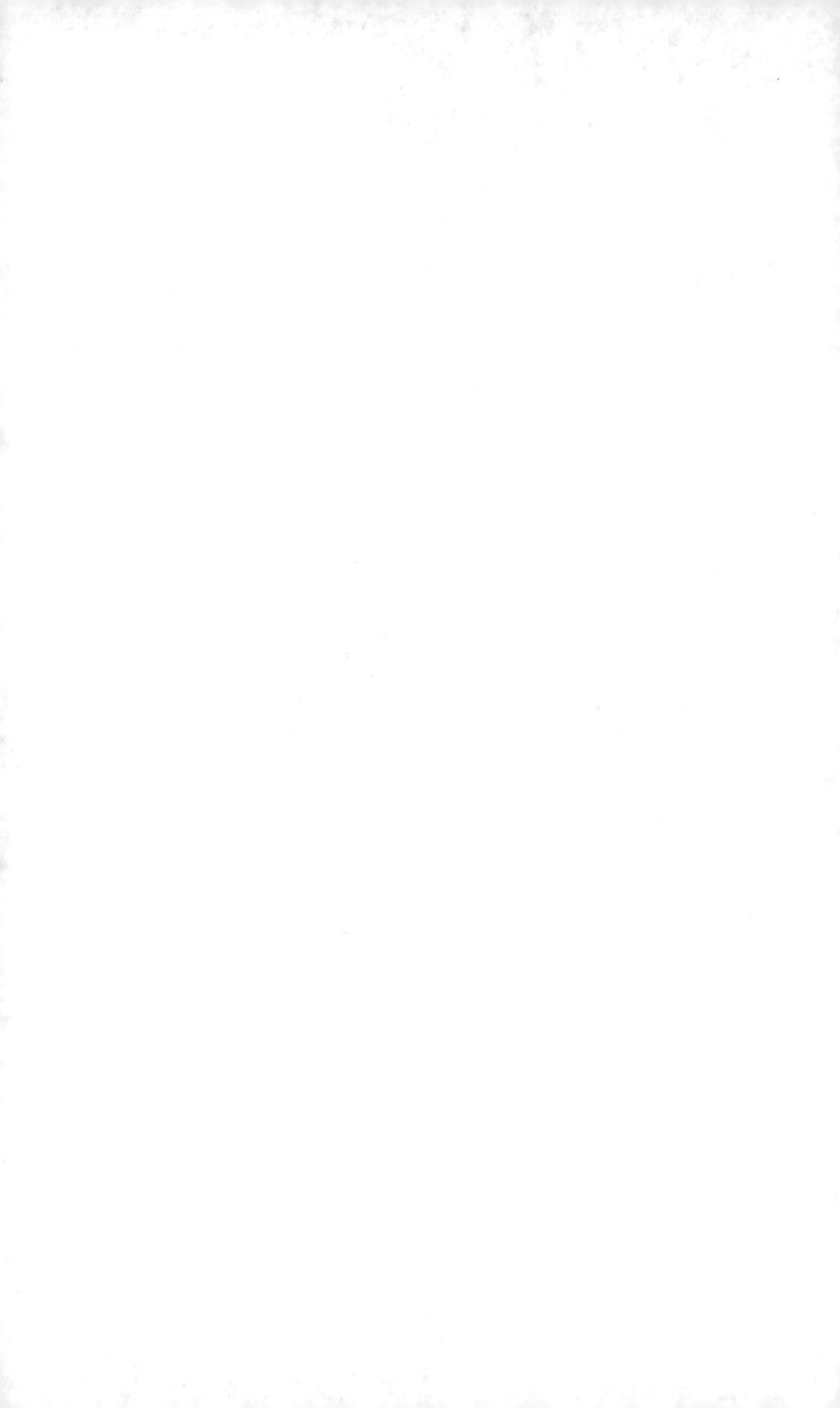

I Can't Sleep, I'm Depressed, *and* I Don't Want a Prescription

Amy Constantine

I Can't Sleep, I'm Depressed,
and I Don't Want a Prescription

Amy Constantine

ISBN-13: 978-1495306952
ISBN-10: 149530695X

"If there's a book
that you want to read,
but it hasn't been written yet,
then you must write it."
~ Toni Morrison

Contact Information
www.anxietyandinsomnia.org

I decided to write this book after having seen so many tragedies in the news related to people suffering from mood disorders. When someone has a kidney problem or appendicitis, no one blames them for their condition. But in our culture, mental illness is whispered about shamefully as if it isn't merely the manifestation of a physical ailment. I felt I needed to share my own experience and insight into how I overcame my sleep and mood issues, and in particular by mostly using natural supplements.

A person's body and experience is unique, of course, but if my story can help somene else in any small way then it will be worth the effort. I hope that by reading my book, you will know that you are not alone in struggling with depression, dread, sleeplessness, or anxiety. I have been there, at the very bottom of the cold lonely barrel, praying and weeping and asking for anything or anyone to help or save me. Never ever give up, even if you do not find the answers here. Believe in yourself and in your value to others. You will make it through this rough time. You have a physical condition, so don't feel ashamed. People who do not suffer from this condition have no idea what is happening to you and how desperate you are to feel better.

I would like to preface this story with a disclaimer that the specific solutions I used are not found in this book. I do not want the responsibility of injuring others, and I make no claims of being a doctor or someone who is licensed or similarly qualified in any capacity. Why write a book then, if not to offer solutions? This book is more of an exploration of my personal journey. It is an informal, nonlinear recollection of what happened to me, and my recommendations are intentionally broad. By sharing my personal journey, I hope that others will find a starting point and be inspired to explore their own options.

Where It All Began: Insomnia

I remember first having problems with insomnia when I was in college. After partying with friends or pulling an all-nighter, a full night's sleep always seemed to elude me. I noted that my friends would quickly crash after a night out, but I would stay awake, staring at the ceiling.

The insomnia wasn't really a major issue until after I got married and had children, in my mid-30s. I chalked my constant sleeplessness up to stress. I also began gaining weight at this time, especially around my mid-section. It was also when I was in my 30s that I noticed I wasn't as outgoing as I was when I was younger. And, after a night of very little sleep, I wasn't able to bounce back the next day like I did when I was younger. Eventually, the thought itself of not being able to sleep gave me a lot of anxiety. My insomnia was also was followed by a mild depression and crabbiness in the morning. The cycle kept repeating itself, driving me to the point of desperation. I tried taking over-the-counter sleeping pills, but these only made me even more tired and depressed the next day.

I recall reading somewhere that people like me who have anxiety generally tend to be smarter and more sensitive or conscientious than others. Very often, we want safety, order, and predictability. We also tend to fret over not only our own problems but take on the worries of others as seriously as our own.

It did not help that on those nights when I couldn't sleep, I would get caught up in the negativity of all the stories on the Internet, such as the failing economy. This overworked my mind, which was already too busy. My thoughts would race, and so would my heart, and I would toss and turn. Then, I learned about the death of a relative who lived far away but was close to my own age. I got anxious about my own nightly heart palpitations, and I began to frantically research health websites, looking for the cause of my perceived heart problems, scared to death by that other death and my own rapid heart-beat. This marked the start of my full-fledged panic attacks. I started checking my blood pressure constantly. My mother had died young from complications related to heart disease and diabetes, so I started to obsessively monitor my blood sugar as well.

This led me to make trip after trip to the hospital emergency room where the doctors were of course all too familiar with nervous women like myself who have been around since the heyday of Sigmund Freud. They humored me, they showed me my normal vital stats, and tried to gently assure me that nothing was wrong.

Unconvinced, I visited two cardiologists. The first put me through a series of unnecessary tests that ran up thousands of dollars in medical bills, only to conclude that I was slightly deficient in Vitamin D.

The other doctor had me wear a heart monitor for a week, put me through a treadmill stress test, and finally made me see that my heart was, in fact, fine. On top of that, I also spent a night in a sleep clinic testing for apnea.

While I continued to see countless other doctors, my mood fluctuated between exhaustion and depression. By then, the panic itself had also extended to attacks in stores while shopping. Movie theaters in particular would send my heart racing and cause shallow breathing. Sitting in the darkness inside the theater, I started to feel that I just might embarrass myself by screaming in panic, with the panic itself caused by the fear of others thinking I was crazy for screaming. The mind really could play tricks on itself, I learned. At that point, I was mostly sleepless at night for fear of insomia itself, and mostly anxious during the day because of panic attacks. I was a wreck.

The panic attacks started to impact on the overall way I related to other people. I had always been shy my entire life, but at that point I started avoiding contact with other people altogether. I just couldn't seem to calm down, relax, just enjoy life, and let things roll off of me anymore. I became impatient, reclusive, and angry, and my whole life revolved around researching on the Internet about what was wrong with me.

I actually hate to blame the Internet for all my problems because in the end, it also helped me find the solutions. However, it had a big part in my downward spiral. Technology certainly made it easy, it helped me in avoiding social interaction: at the self-checkout line at the grocery store, for example, and texting people instead of calling them. No doubt about it, machines definitely help and conspire with the avoidant person in minimizing real, human contact with other people.

I certainly had to go through what I went through to finally learn, later, that the only way out of panic was through it. The more you avoid people and situations, the worse your fear of them becomes. It's like a monster that keeps growing the more you try not to look at it. The only was to slay that monster is to deal with it head on: go straight to the heart of your fear and confront it.

The Doctors

While I did have the misfortune of running into a few bad doctors, there were several along the way who tried to help and gave me some clues about what was wrong with me.

I went to see a well-known chiropractor who charged hundreds of dollars per session and was regarded as a miracle worker by people I knew. In the end, her method involved swallowing large amounts of Omega 3 fish oils. Hmm, there was a clue. I dismissed her as a quack at the time but later I was to learn that she knew part of the answer to my problems.

I also went to see an herbalist who recommended herbs to help calm me, and getting off of coffee and artificial sweeteners. There was also a doctor of Chinese medicine who hinted that I had problems with low estrogen and digestion and said I needed more "heat" in my system and spicy food. Another, very kind doctor tested my hormones and did further blood tests and again noted that everything was normal except for a Vitamin D deficiency and borderline anemia . . . even more clues. Yet another doctor chose to focus on my acid reflux and found that I had a urinary tract infection for which he prescribed antibiotics.

I was starting to see that there were problems with not only my mood but with my body's ability to absorb necessary nutrients and vitamins. I found that while I was not yet diabetic, my body was having difficulty metabolizing sugar and I was headed down the road to diabetes. This discovery only added to my anxiety and health phobias. On top of all of this, I was losing my hair, and constantly running to the bathroom to urinate. I lost 50 pounds in 3 months. All this does not even begin to include how horrible my moods were with my family.

Counseling

Desperate for relief, I sought the help of a psychologist for some counseling. I paid about 12 visits to her, and it was indeed educational. She was the one who helped me see the causes of my panic attacks, and the need to do exactly what it was that I feared, multiple times, until the discomfort went away.

I studied some psychology in college, so I understood how when people are scared of spiders, for example, they gradually have to move in small steps towards actually touching a spider. However, this knowledge was of no consolation to me when I sat inside a movie theater, or was in social situations, wanting to flee. Still, soldier on I did. I kept pushing through all my fears repeatedly until they eventually disappeared.

Wanting To Be Happy

At the most basic level, in order to recover from these problems, even before any type of intervention, I had to convince myself that I wanted to get better, I had reasons to be alive, I had goals, and I had to let go of fear. Worriers and goal-oriented control freaks are somewhat valued in the modern world, and up until that point I always felt that fear and obsessiveness had served me well. Controlling all the variables in my life was the key to my success! But when life gets messy, as it sometimes does, it dawns on you that all that worry won't pay the bills or keep loved ones alive. I had to let myself let go of the fear, and my need for security that motivated all my actions. I needed to appreciate the here and now. Obviously, I wasn't driving the roller coaster, so I should learn to sit back and enjoy the ride. Some people call this "learning to let go," others call it "letting go and letting God." Whatever the avenue, my first step was to throw my hands up in the air and say to myself that I didn't care.

I was once in a skate shop and I said to the salesperson, "You skaters have a lot in common with snowboarders."

"We are all alike, skaters, surfers, snowboarders . . . we all have an appreciation for nature and its resources and for the earth. And we are all very Zen, we go with the flow."

"I am not one of you," I said. "I am a control freak and am only now, at this late stage in my life, learning how to just go with it."

"At least you are learning. Some people never learn."

Indeed, zen master. Indeed.

Prescription Medication

I then opted to do what most people in my position would have done much earlier, which was to try prescription medications. My brief foray into the world of antidepressants and pharmaceuticals was short-lived. I hemmed and hawed for a very long time before deciding to try an antidepressant, and I do not judge those that they have helped and continue to help. Naturally, being the overthinker that I am, I did a great deal of online research before trying pills. I combed through hundreds of reviews of all the various drugs and saw that some people swore by them, while others' lives were destroyed by either their side effects such as liver or sexual dysfunction or withdrawal when trying to wean themselves off the pills.

I was scared, but the pain of my depression and anxiety had gotten so bad that I was willing to try anything. Finally, I set up an appointment to get some medication. The psychiatrist did not try to dissuade me, he just looked at me with jaded eyes, surprised that I waited as long as I did given that there was no need to suffer. He put me on a mild antidepressant and Klonopin to help me fall into a regular sleep cycle.

My system is very sensitive to medication and after a few days of walking around feeling like a zombie, I decided that pharmaceuticals were not for me. Granted, I did not wait the recommended amount of time, something like 4 weeks, for the pills to realize their maximum effectiveness. And, it was also very nice to feel numb to all my problems.

In the end, it was a personal decision on my part not to go back to drugs. I have also fought to avoid antidepressants. It has not been an easy road but I just feel it was the best for me. One of the last things my mother said to me in her dying days was to try to avoid any chemical solutions that the doctors give you. Those words have stayed with me through all my struggle.

Digestion and Thyroid

I believe that the causes of depression are two fold. First, the food we eat is less nutrient rich than it used to be, and that antibiotics and germs have compromised our digestive tracts' ability to break down and unlock what few nutrients are in left our food. Because we can't get vitamins out of our food, our health, and our mental health in particular, suffers. Second, the germs and lack of vitamins, when mixed with many people's overreliance on stimulants, cause our poor pituitary and thyroid glands to go haywire.

Several websites run by people like me who have found their own answers talk about how doctors in this country are not equipped to properly test for thyroid problems. Online, (where yes, many things are untrue) they say that one way you can get around a false "everything is fine" thyroid test is to measure your basal body temperature when you first wake up. If it is low, there may be a chance that you have a sluggish thyroid gland. I don't know whether this is true, but I tested myself and found my body temperature to be alarmingly low each time I would wake up.

What Do I Do?

I went through all the regular medical channels and still nothing was working. I was still sleepless and always on the verge of a nervous breakdown and had to take matters into my own hands because no one could help me.

How Did I Get Better?

There is no quick and easy answer to that question. I will say that at my worst, on a scale from 1 to 10, my depression and anxiety was at an 11. I was about to throw away my entire family, my career, my friends, and had no reason to want to continue to live. Today, I can honestly rate my mood problems on a daily basis to be between 3 and 5. This may not seem like a successful outcome to some people, but for me it is a huge victory.

I would rate my insomnia, also once quite severe, at about a 4. I still do not sleep like a baby, getting between 5 and 7 hours of occasionally broken sleep per night but I do not take pills and I do not feel tired the next day. I used to worry about not getting the recommended 8 to10 hours of sleep at night, but then I heard a sleep expert on TV say that the amount of sleep each person needs varies. Some people can get by on 3 hours, others need 10. How much you yawn the next day is the biggest indicator of whether or not you are getting enough sleep.

Today, my hair is no longer falling out, my acid reflux is gone, and I am no longer urinating frequently. My urinary tract infections are no more, my weight is normal, and the blood sugar stays at low levels.

My personal solution came from me using my own resources to experiment with natural supplements and using myself as a guinea pig. Following my "gut" instinct that something was wrong with my gut, I took plant supplements and probiotics that are said to kill the candida and *H.pylori* virus in the intestinal tract. I can't be certain that there is anything to this idea either, but after making these changes I did start to gain weight again and I felt like food was moving through my system again. I found that contrary to popular belief, digestion is not about having too much acid (HCL) in your stomach, it is about having too little. When you do not have enough acid down there, the food sits in your intestinal tract and cannot be broken down to be used effectively by the body.

Blood Sugar and Diabetes

I read about diabetes, and I found that the cur rent medical standard for what is regarded as normal blood sugar will eventually cause the disease to progress and organ damage to occur. In reality, blood sugar should be kept at between 80 and110 all day long (see Dr. Richard Bernstein's *Diabetes*

Solution). I tried veganism, I tried high protein diets. The only thing that has worked for me is eating about a playing-card-deck portion size of protein, and one cup of green vegetables per meal, about every 4 hours, per Dr. Bernstein. Without going into all of the detail here, mood and urination is impacted by changes in blood sugar and the best course of action is to try to keep your blood sugar low and steady, minimizing fluctuations when possible. Simple carbohydrates are the diabetic's main enemy.

Going After the Two Big Problems

Next, with my body better able to digest, I decided to tackle my two biggest problems: Mood and Insomnia. Again, I honestly think that both mood and insomnia are related to hormonal and thyroid problems caused by poor nutrition and absorption. Hormones also play a role. I consider depression and anxiety to be partners in crime or two sides of the same card. If your energy is low, worries will crop up. In a nutshell, you have to have the right balance of energy and calmness AND estrogen and testosterone to be in the right zone, mentally and physically. And if you are not getting enough vitamins, B vitamins in particular, through diet, you need to take supplements.

The good news is that nature gives us the keys to control energy and calmness, and plants can help us moderate estrogen and testosterone. Everything that we put on our skin and in our bloodstream prompts an almost immediate physical and mental reaction, usually within 10 to 30 minutes. So I would pay close attention to what would happen after taking a certain pill or eating certain foods. There are things in nature that will speed you up like "uppers" while other things are "downers."

When I first tried to attack my paralyzing anxiety, I mistakenly thought to just throw everything but the kitchen sink into calming myself down, so I over-loaded on "downers." I am nervous, I thought, so I better do some things to calm myself down. Naturally, I became more depressed, sluggish, listless, and weepy until I finally made the following brilliant statement to my husband, "Here's something I learned the hard way: Too many downers will bring you down!"

I haven't figured it all out, but I get the sense that mood is all related to the liver. Whenever I have coffee or alcohol, or anything bitter, I can feel my liver move. For some reason I get the sense that the liver holds estrogen, which affects energy. Whenever you take something that stimulates the liver, changes in mood and energy take place.

The key is balancing energy and calmness, and my personal solution was to take natural stimulants in the morning, including those that would nourish my thyroid and taking calmatives at night to help me sleep. You can't go too far in either direction, otherwise mood problems will develop. Sometimes, depression and panic develop from your body not having the juice to move the liver and digestion, and you need uppers. But if you are too stimulated, the body fearfully contracts your muscles and stomach, and won't move food through your tract. Caffeine is a good and obvious example. Just like cocaine, cocoa, amphetamines, or anything that is known to rev you up, too many stimulants of any kind cause aggressiveness and irritability. How much stimulation any person will need will again, like sleep, depend on that person. I once read an interview with the comedian Robin Williams where he said that he used to use cocaine to "bring him down."

The trick is to find the balance point in your system and to know which stimulating supplements help you get to that balance point. Over and again, I would read in the review sections of certain supplements that what works for one person may be completely ineffective for another.

The advantage in using natural supplements seems to be fewer side effects, which is not to say they don't have any. Just because it is natural doesn't make it safe. I had many terrible supplements that did not agree with my body causing tremendous mood swings.

Estrogen Versus Testosterone: An Epic Battle

A similar approach needs to be taken when finding the right balance between estrogen and testosterone. Both pharmaceuticals and natural supplements can impact that balance point. I have to come to a better understanding of where I need to be to be happy and that is to run a little heavier on the testosterone side.

When I took too many plant supplements known to increase estrogen, my problems worsened dramatically. Looking back now, I see that my estrogen levels were probably too high. A lot of reviews will tell women that our estrogen levels decrease as we age, and this is true, but you don't want to push estrogen too high because I believe estrogen is already plentiful in the plastics we use and the meat we consume. My only unscientific measure for estrogen is my own guessing and intuition. When I have a lot of estrogen in my system I start to: bake more for my family, I hug them more, I will put on more makeup, and change my earrings to match my clothes. My skin feels softer and lips look fuller. I am happier and more creative and wear brighter colors. I clean the house more and feel like decorating when I'm full of estrogen.

But too much estrogen will also bring out panic attacks, cause emotionally charged and weepy fights with my husband, frequent urination, my hair to fall out more, swelling, brain fog, and cold hands and feet. Excess estrogen also makes me more sedentary and will raise my blood sugar. Mayonnaise, for example, which contains soy, seems to cause all of the aforementioned symptoms, whenever I have too much of it.

I also experimented with using food and supplements to lower my estrogen and raise my testosterone and when I did I noticed the following symptoms: Increased facial hair growth, aggressiveness, amazing energy, rapid heartbeat, disappearance of frequent urination, being more driven and goal oriented, a deepening of the voice, not cooking or cleaning as much for my family, not feeling as caring or loving, not as funny and creative, wearing more pants and darker colors, heck, even taking up carpentry! When I was feeling manly in this way, all my panic disappeared completely and interestingly, too much testosterone would again increase my blood sugar.

As with taking too many stimulants or too much estrogen, too much testosterone was also bad, giving me symptoms commonly associated with "roid rage." I'd become irritable, impatient, domineering and angry. I was like a bulldozer. However, if you are somehow able to find that right balance between estrogen and testosterone, voila, all problems including mood, libido and sleep related problems, magically disappear! Libido in particular only comes about when that perfect balance is achieved.

Clearly, nature aims for balance and variety. In summary, when exploring supplements:

1. Heal your digestive tract. There are probiotics, digestive enzymes and germ killers that will help you get your system absorbing vitamins from food again. Explore the possibility that you might have a problem with your thyroid gland.

2. Take multivitamins. Strong ones. Vitamin C and Vitamins B are the most important of all. In my mind, Vitamin B or the lack thereof, is the key to depression.

3. You need energy in the morning, and lots of it. But if you have too much, and feel yourself becoming aggressive, you need to take whatever works for you to calm yourself down. But not too calm! Experiment with plant supplements that help moderate energy versus calm to get to the point where you are comfortable and alert. And at night you need to find the plants that will knock you out cold so that you can sleep.

4. Estrogen and testosterone need to be in balance. Look at the list of symptoms above. If you are experiencing any of those symptoms, you have too many hormones in one direction or another and need to find a balance using supplements.

Final
Thoughts

While I am uncertain what it was that caused me to get sick (my guess is that it was and is bacteria and being exposed to too much estrogen), I would not for a minute take back what I learned throughout my hellish odyssey. Illness helped me to understand the importance of being in the moment, loving me for me and gave me a tremendous empathy for others in the same situation. It made me want to help others.

Once you are in balance and get a second chance at life, you are more grateful. Illness makes you re-evaluate your direction. Having gotten myself more physically in balance, I have come to see that I needed to let go of certain feelings and ideas that were shackling me, stop worrying about the future and go out and talk to people more. I now purposely try, once per day, to do something that scares me.

Once I felt healthier and more confident and assertive, I started to concoct dreams again, and set goals that made me happy. A large part of depression is not being true to yourself and not pursuing what it is that makes your heart happy. You have to be in pursuit of something or be at work on a project you feel is worthwhile, to connect with your soul. Once you go out to do this, the money will fall into place. You have to believe in you and your own greatness.

I will make one very specific recommendation, apart from Dr. Bernstein's book: please read *The Woman's Guide to Having It All* by Celia Ward Wallace. It is a simple instructional manual of sorts on how to teach yourself to be happy. Finally, if you would like to contact me, you may go to the website www. anxietyandinsomnia.org. Good luck in your own personal journey. You *will* make it!